GET OUTTA My HEAD

MY JOURNEY LIVING WITH BRAIN CANCER

COLLETTE A. HENRY

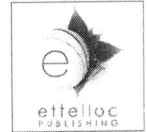

Cover design, interior book design and eBook design
by Blue Harvest Creative
www.blueharvestcreative.com

Get Outta My Head
Copyright © 2013 Collette A. Henry
All rights reserved. This book or any portion thereof may not be reproduced or used in any manner whatsoever without the express written permission of the publisher except for the use of brief quotations in a book review.

Printed in the United States of America
First Printing 2013

Published by
Ettelloc Publishing
734 Franklin Avenue, Suite #235
Garden City, NY 11530

ISBN-13: 978-0615786223
ISBN-10: 0615786227
LCCN: 2013935367

"Cancer may have started the fight, but I will finish it."
~ gotcancer.org ~

Table of Contents

7
FOREWORD
Allen O. Green

13
CHAPTER ONE
Doing What I Love

19
CHAPTER TWO
My Surgeries

30
CHAPTER THREE
My Cancer

36
CHAPTER FOUR
My Life Before Cancer

50
CHAPTER FIVE
Cancer Can Hit Anyone

58
CHAPTER SIX
Fallout and Treatments

66
CHAPTER SEVEN
Who Am I?

70
CHAPTER EIGHT
Life Goes On

Acknowledgements

I'd like to take a moment to recognize my parents and my siblings for all the support they gave me throughout this period in my life. I love you dearly.

Foreword
By Allen O. Green

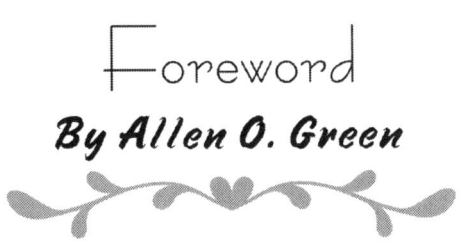

LIFE IS UNPREDICTABLE; we never know what it will throw our way. It is a topsy-turvy, roller-coaster ride that has exhilarating highs and distressing, crushing lows. It is an amalgamation of positive and negative experiences. When we face the good, we do so without much effort for it does not disturb the general flow of how we live. It does not call for much mental, emotional and physical effort to embrace what is pleasant. After all, any changes in this area is for the better.

Conversely, when unpleasant things occur, every facet of our beings is distorted and in many instances, we lose hope and feel as if we cannot endure what life has cast. How we react to what life brings us our way determines in many cases how we live the remainder of our days, particularly when the occurrence of negative life events and adversities come our way. Well, the story Collette has written is one that shows us how to stand up to those unexpected curveballs that comes our way at times and knock them out of the park!

I have been friends with Collette for a number of years and I must acknowledge that I met her just following the majority of the events detailed in this book. I cannot speak on the episodes that transpired in this text but I can speak to the individual that rose out of the ashes of adversity.

My friend Collette can be defined in many constructive ways; words such as bright, sunny, optimistic and fearless come to mind. However, one of the things that really catch my attention is her stubbornness. When I say stubborn, I am speaking of the term in a positive light in this instance. From what I witnessed during our friendship and from what I have read in this work, I can emphatically say that she stubbornly stared cancer in the face and refused to allow this disease to take her life or change her outlook on it.

Whenever I recall all that she endured and overcame during that period, I am taken aback and wonder if I could ever face such challenges and bounce back in the fashion that she did. When Collette decided to write her story about that tumultuous time and I read the manuscript, my respect for her grew even more and her story inspires hope in me during my dark days when life is not so compassionate.

In reading Collette's journey, you will see how brain cancer not only affected her life upon its discovery but you will see the far-reaching ramifications that affects not only her future but also how it affected her past. That being said, Collette pierces the veil of her own life in order to show us that receiving a diagnosis of brain cancer is not the end, but it can be a beginning - a beginning where you can honestly look back on your life and assess how every life event in your past has prepared you for whatever you may face today!

Collette never uses her cancer as a scapegoat to blame all her life decisions on - whether they were good or bad. She recognizes it for what it is, viz. cancer is an aspect of her life that affected it but has not ruled it. She candidly shares with her readers many things that most would never acknowledge publicly let alone write in a book. In addition, Collette appreciatively acknowledges that she could not have done this without the love and support of others.

It is my fondest hope that you benefit greatly from reading the account of how my friend faced brain cancer with the contagious, bright and cheery smile that she carries with her everywhere she goes and appreciate that when it was all said and done, she is still smiling.

*Dedicated to Allen O. Green
for helping me to see this book to completion.*

Chapter One
Doing what I love

> *"Running is the greatest metaphor for life, because you get out of it what you put into it....This is the hardest thing there is for me. Nothing is harder - work, accomplishments, achievements - than the actual mental and physical discipline that it takes to do this. But this is what I have to do to get the kind of mental and physical sharpness that I want."*
> ~ Oprah Winfrey ~

BUTTERFLIES IN MY stomach - I usually get this way before the start of every race. That day was no exception.

The day was Wednesday, May 20, 2009. It was a regular workday like any other typical workday for me. Five o'clock came, signaling the end of the workday. I went into the ladies room to change from my work clothes into my running gear. After I finished changing, I looked in the mirror one last time and took a deep breath. Then, after I met up with members of our company's running team, we traveled on the subway together to Central Park in Manhattan where the race would begin.

We arrived at the meet up location - Tavern on the Green - and we put our bags on a nearby bench. Then as usual, we started to do a warm-up run. My run was a little longer than most of the other runners that day. After our warm up, we all started to stretch our muscles to loosen up.

The tension in my stomach was getting stronger as race time approached. I now felt a beating in my chest. Five minutes to go, and we headed to the starting line. We all got in our last minute stretching as we waited for the sound of the gun to go off for the race to begin. It seemed like an eternity, but finally the signal was given and we took off.

As a rule of thumb, I generally start running slow to regulate my pace. That day, I started out slow and was running side by side with a member of my own team. We were feeding off of each other's pace, making sure to keep up with the other. I could almost hear his breathing match my own. Things were going smoothly. I was running at a fairly good pace, thanks to my teammate!

Then, about 2 miles into the race, I stopped - dead in my tracks. All I remember is my head was spinning and I had turned around in the opposite direction. (I was later told that I was spinning in circles, and hopping on one leg before falling to the ground.)

Get outta my head!

The next thing I knew, I woke up in an unfamiliar environment. It took me a moment to realize I was in an ambulance. I looked up at the technician, still dazed. He asked me if I knew what happened - I was too disoriented to respond. He told me that I had a seizure. I didn't fully understand what he was telling me, since I was just beginning to regain consciousness.

While lying down on the gurney in the ambulance, I looked up and saw my team members. I don't recall what I said to them. Then I noticed my mouth felt funny while I was speaking. At some point while I had my seizure, my capped tooth had fallen out. So there I was, at first, unbeknownst to me, talking without a front tooth. As soon as I realized this, I covered my mouth with my hand in embarrassment whenever I spoke to anyone.

At this point the ambulance was ready to take me to the hospital, so one of my team members gave the technician my belongings and we drove off. They took me to St. Luke's-Roosevelt Hospital in Manhattan.

I don't remember the ambulance ride or even getting to the hospital. I didn't even recall being taken to my room. Most of my hospital stay was a big blur.

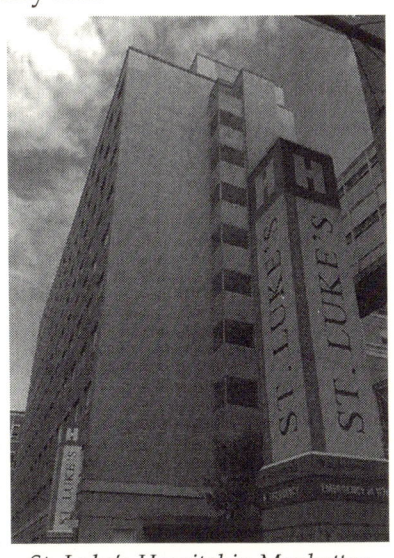

St. Luke's Hospital in Manhattan

Once at the hospital, the first person I called was my younger brother Aqiyl. He rushed to the hospital. Medical staff was abuzz, coming in and out of my room. I was taken for a CT scan and an MRI so that the doctors could see more of what was going on in my head.

After many tests, it was revealed that I had a tumor in my brain. I wondered ...

How I got a brain tumor?
How did a simple seizure turn into a something like that, since people have seizures every day?

Honestly, looking back, I really didn't know much about seizures or tumors at that point. I heard of people having seizures, but I didn't know that seizures were an indication of my current condition.

Once hearing this, my brother Aqiyl called my parents who live in Florida. Word started getting around and immediately my family and friends started to arrive at the hospital.

When people started to come to visit me, I was still self-conscious about my missing front tooth. So I would cover my mouth with my hand when they first saw me. I would explain to them that my front tooth fell out, and then I would remove my hand from the front of my face. To my surprise, no one gasped in horror. They just shook it off, and asked me "why are you worrying about that at a time like this?"

Everyone wondered how this could happen to me. I was physically fit. Just as this was a big question for them, it was an even bigger question for me since I was the one experiencing it. But I just let the end result sink in. I had a tumor. I'm sure that the thought of cancer was running through people's minds upon hearing this, including me.

I know that some people at this point would have been angry and said to their tumor, "Who invited to you into my head?" They would have wanted to be able to get rid of the tumor with just their bare hands.

I think most people facing what I was dealing with goes through the 5 stages of grief. The 1st stage is **denial**. This is where they'd say, "I'm fine, this can't be happening to me." This is where a person just refuses to face facts or the reality and severity of the situation.

Then they would transition to the 2nd stage which is **anger**. This is where an individual might demand answers to questions like "Why me?" and "Who is to blame?" They may also say things like "It's not fair." Some people can be angry with themselves, or with others, and especially those who are close to them.

Then the 3rd stage is **bargaining**. This is where someone might say things like, "I'll do anything for a few more years;" "I will give my life savings for more time". This is where people have hope that they can postpone or delay death.

After bargaining comes **depression**, the 4th stage. This is where one might say things like "I'm so sad, why bother with anything?" "I'm going to die soon so what's the point?" "I will miss my loved one, why go on?" The person may try to disconnect themselves from loved ones. It's natural to feel sadness, regret, fear, and uncertainty when going through this stage.

The last and 5th stage of grief is **acceptance**. This is where a person might say things like, "It's going to be okay;" "I can't fight it, I may as well prepare for it." People in this stage have come to terms with their mortality or tragic events.

Strangely enough, I bypassed all 4 and landed on the 5th stage which is acceptance.

Returning to my story, one of my doctors came into my room to speak with me about what the next steps were. He said that I needed to have a biopsy done to determine if the tumor was benign (non-cancerous), or malignant (cancerous). I said fine.

He then left my room to consult with his medical team. He came back in and told me that though they initially wanted to just do a biopsy, he now had an alternate solution that he wanted to run by me.

He said that the tumor, whether cancerous or not, did not belong in my head, so he wanted to perform major surgery to remove the tumor, because it was pressing against parts of my brain. I said okay, since in my mind that actually did seem like the most logical route to go, and I was prepared to say good riddance to my tumor.

Get outta my head!

I later learned that the skull is only meant to house three things, the brain, blood vessels and cerebrospinal fluid, so my tumor was an unwelcome mass taking up space in my head.

Chapter Two
My surgeries

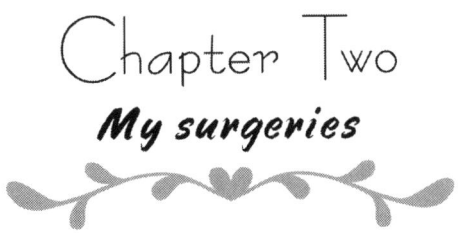

"Why do you think it is (commonly held)..." I asked Dr. Cook... "that brain surgery, above all else - even rocket science - gets singled out as the most challenging of human feats, the one demanding the utmost of human intelligence?" [Dr. Cook answered] "No margin for error."
~ Michael J. Fox ~

SURGERY DAY HAD finally arrived! It was May 26, 2009. I had been in the hospital for almost one week before surgery day. The medical staff had to do blood workups, and generally monitored me during this time period. They asked questions regarding any allergies to medications that I had, which up to this point I had none.

The day of my surgery, my neurosurgeon came to talk to me about the procedure that was going to take place. Before the surgery itself, they would shave part of my hair to ensure that the area was clean. They would then perform a craniotomy, where an incision would be made in my skull to remove the bone flap. Then the tumor would be removed and the bone flap put back in place secured by titanium clips. Once the bone was replaced, the incision would be closed with staples.

He then asked me if I had any questions or concerns, and I said no. So, I was wheeled off to the operating room. Then the anesthesiologist told me that she was going to put the mask over my mouth and nose and that I should count back down starting from 10. I barely recall saying 10.

The next thing I knew I woke up in the recovery room. Once the staff realized that I was awake, they came in to take my vitals and ask me if I was alright. I was desperately in need of getting something for my pain - after all, I had just had my head cut open.

My neurosurgeon came to check up on me. He told me that the operation went well. However, they only removed the bulk of the tumor. The residual piece was resting on my motor cortex so they could not remove that portion. If they did, I could have been left paralyzed on the right side of my body.

After receiving the pain medication, I fell back asleep and when I woke up, I saw that my family and my ex-husband, Rod, were there. I was so happy to see them all. I saw the mixed emotions in some of their faces. They were happy and relieved that I made it through the surgery; but they still looked worried.

I think the severity of the event hit them when they saw the blood seepage bag coming from under my head bandage that was there to capture the residual blood flowing out from beneath my incision.

They stayed as long as they could, until it was time for the medical staff to tend to me, so then they left. The staff duties included getting me ready for a sponge bath. I thought I'd be embarrassed since this was the first time receiving a sponge bath, but I was sort of sedated, so I didn't care.

I was then moved from the recovery room into my semi private room. My roommate was a woman who had just had her 7th brain operation, and she seemed to be in just as good spirits as I was. We were both just taking it in stride.

So, here I am, starting to welcome more of my visitors. People from my job, my gym, college, my track team members, and of course my family came on a regular basis. So many people brought gifts, flowers, food, you name it, and they brought it. One of my relatives even gave me a coloring book to pass the time. I thought that was such a cute idea.

Most days were blurry, but some days I could recall what was going on, and one day in particular stood out. That was when my track coach, Mr. Pope, came to visit me. I was so caught off guard and we both had tears in our eyes. I think the sight of me reminded him of the brain issues that he himself had. We went into the visitors lounge and he stayed with me for quite a while. We talked about my college days on the track team, and he kept me updated on current events in the track arena.

My gal pal team (Genny, Marsha, and LaVerne) was also consistently visiting me in the hospital. I truly appreciated this because I knew they were traveling from great distances to visit with me. I recall one time Marsha was on her way out to see me. She got into a car accident on the highway. After getting that all straightened out, she could have just turned around and gone home and given me a call to check up on me, but instead she continued with the long drive just to see me in person. That gesture meant so much to me.

I recall one day, I had a seizure. Next thing I was aware of, I came to and hospital staff was on top of me doing chest compressions. I told my friends about it. They looked at each other, and then looked at me. They said to me, you know what that means? Your heart must have stopped. I was so drugged up that I didn't even comprehend it at the moment.

My mom spent many nights in the hospital with me. I'm not a parent, but I can only imagine how devastating it must be to watch your child go through brain surgery or any kind of traumatic experience. Not only was it physically uncomfortable for her to sleep in a chair to be with me, I'm sure that it was emotionally draining on her part to watch me go through what I was facing.

Anytime I had visitors, I truly felt the sincerity in their voices when they said "let me know if there is anything I can do for you". I'll forever be in the debt to my family and friends for everything they did for me during my time of need.

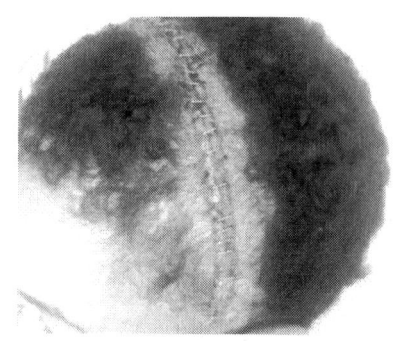
My surgical scar

Then it was time for my bandages to come off. My anticipation at seeing my scar began to rise. Once they were off, I looked in the mirror and saw the tremendous scar that ran from almost ear to ear. I was more intrigued than shocked at the sight.

Finally, it was time to be discharged. My mom and I spent the first week of my recovery at my sister Toni's home. Before we got there, my mom and I stopped off at my apartment so that I could gather some of my belongings. If felt so good to be back in my own home, even though it was just for a few minutes. I packed a small suitcase and we headed to my sister's place. Some friends and family came to visit me during this week and they were a pleasant sight for sore eyes.

While my sister went to work, my mom would cook breakfast for me. Then after that I basically stayed in my sister's home office on the computer playing around on Facebook and watching television. Then when my sister came home from work, my mom would cook dinner for the three of us. This was our basic routine for a week.

As I was home recovering, about one week later, I woke up and my left eye was partially swollen shut. I knew something was terribly wrong. I immediately called my father so that he could take me to the hospital. He called my brother Aqiyl who met us there. By the time we arrived, my left eye was completely shut.

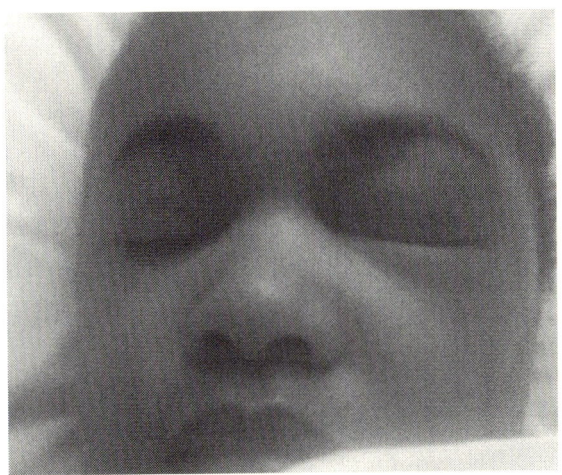

Effect of the brain infection

My brother and I went into the emergency room while my father found parking. Inside with my brother, I knew that I'd have to just wait my turn, but he impatiently insisted on bringing me up to the front desk for them to admit me immediately. The attendant told him that I needed to fill out a form and just wait my turn.

Once it was my turn, I was taken to a room for observation. The medical staff quickly realized that they would have to readmit me. Once they did, the doctors immediately started to run all kinds of tests to determine what was wrong.

It turned out I had some type of infection in my brain. The infectious disease specialist had to be called in to make sure it was not something contagious. I was quarantined for a little while, but it turned out that it wasn't anything transmittable.

So, **once** again, my neurosurgeon came in to speak with me. He informed me that I would need another surgery to remove the infection.

The procedure was basically the same as the first surgery, except this time they were removing the infection and not another part of my tumor.

After the surgery I woke up in such severe agony that I was actually crying. The staff asked me to rate my pain on a scale of 1 to 10. I told them it was a 10 and they gave me medication for it. Looking back, I would have rated my initial surgery a 4 compared to what I experienced after the second surgery.

I was in so much pain that I begged God to take my life. But then I was given morphine and once it kicked in, all was well.

Because of the infection, I had to have a PICC line surgically inserted into my upper arm to do self-administered antibiotic treatments. A PICC line is a Peripherally Inserted Central Catheter, which is a long, slender, small, flexible tube inserted into a vein in my upper arm. The tube travels in my arm, up to a vein in the chest near my heart.

The PICC line was inserted and then I was released that same day. I was sent home with a hand-full of prescriptions for medications that I needed to start taking that night.

This time, my mother and I stayed with my brother Aqiyl, at my parent's home that they kept in Queens. By the time we arrived, it was nearing nighttime. Since my brother had to go to work the next day, my mom drove me to get my prescriptions filled.

The first pharmacy that we went to didn't have the medications on hand. We drove around looking for another all night pharmacy, but couldn't find one. I called my ex-husband to see if he could give us directions to a pharmacy, and luckily he was able to direct us to one. We got there and put in the order to fill my prescriptions. We then had to wait about an hour before all my medications were filled. Then we made our way back home for what seemed to have taken forever.

I had so many medications to take, and at different times, so I had to create a chart detailing when, how much to take, and even how to finally wean myself off some of them. After all this, I was able to take my medications for the night, and I was then finally able to go to bed.

The next day, a home care nurse came out in the morning to show me how to self-administer my antibiotics. She brought with her an I.V. pole and the medication bags. They were filled with antibiotics and she told me that they were to be refrigerated until a few hours before it was time to administer them.

She also showed me how to clean the PICC line using alcohol pads. She swabbed the tip of the PICC line with one of the pads. She removed the cap from one of the antibiotic bags, hung it from the I.V. pole, connected it to the tubing, and then attached it the PICC line in my arm. Then she opened the airway in the tubing and the liquids started to flow.

After the bag was completely finished, she closed the airway from the I.V. pole and disconnected it from the tubing in my PICC line. She then asked me if I had any questions. I said no.

My mother and brother were there in the room watching the entire procedure with me, so in case I was hesitant about something, I'd be able to get reassurance from them. Then she left me with a week's supply of antibiotics, wished me well, and then went on her way. Each week, I received a new shipment in the mail of antibiotics for a month and a half.

I had to self-administer twice a day, and since the nurse did my morning dosage, it was now my turn to do my evening dosage. I waited until my brother came home from work, and then between him and my mother, we were ready to give it a try.

Neither of them really wanted me to do it on my own, so we all took part in the procedure, each person doing one part of the process. When it was time to open the line so that the fluids would flow through, it didn't work at first, but on the second try it started to flow down into my arm. It was a relief to see that it was actually working, because I was alarmed when I didn't see it functioning properly at first.

The next day, a different nurse came out just to ensure that I was performing the process properly. He watched as I did it on my own, and he said that I did everything correctly. I was still a little nervous, but slowly getting the hang of it.

The morning dosage was fine. But the evening dosage was the most trying time for me. Not because it was difficult to administer, but because of all the liquids being poured into my body, I kept getting up during the night to use the bathroom.

The next day, my mother drove me back to my home so that I could gather some more clothes, since it seemed as though I'd be staying at my brother's place for a few months while I recovered.

Before returning home, we made a pit stop. I needed something to cover the PICC line. There was a piece of tubing that was dangling from my arm that I wanted to cover up. So we went to a store and I bought a pair of leg warmers. I cut the length in half and used it to cover the PICC line whenever I went out in public.

So now we're back at my brothers and it's time for me to move from where I was sleeping at first, which was the couch, into the basement bedroom. My brother cleared out all of his belongings from the room, I unpacked my clothes and then I made myself at home.

During the following few days, I was still receiving gifts, especially from people at my job. I received flower arrangements, fruit baskets, chocolates, and assortments of little trinkets. I almost thought that we would run out of places to put all the gifts.

During the next several weeks, I had many visitors. One of the things they mentioned was that they could not believe that I underwent brain surgery. They thought that I would be confined to my bed.

During the initial days and weeks, I had various doctor appointments. I had to meet with my family doctor, my oncologist, and my neurologist. My mother drove me to most of them, and sometimes my brother would take off from work to take me other appointments.

Then finally, the 6 weeks of taking my antibiotics was over. I thought that I was going to have to go back to the hospital to have my PICC line removed, but a home care nurse came to the house to remove it. I thought it was going to be a big to do, but she basically just pulled the string right out from my upper arm. Then she just put a band aide on the area and I was good as new.

What wasn't good as new was my sleep pattern. A carryover from being in the hospital was my lack of sleep. While in the hospital I was consistently being awakened every few hours for nurses to check my vital signs and things of that nature. This irregular sleep pattern still affects me to this day.

I went to my primary care physician regarding my lack of sleep, and he prescribed Ambien. The first two nights taking it, I had disturbing nightmares. The first night I dreamt that I was being chased down to be raped. The next night I dreamt that family members were going to be murdered.

There were far worse effects to the Ambien than the nightmares. I started having memory lapses. One night I recall that I was watching television, propped up on two pillows and I was wearing my eyeglasses. The next thing I knew, I woke up in the middle of the night, the television was off, one of the pillows was removed and my eyeglasses were in its case.

I could not recall doing any of these things the night before. That was the last time that I took the Ambien. My memory is bad enough without me taking a medication to make it even worse. In light of all this, I'd rather just suffer through insomnia.

After about 2 months at my brother's place, I decided I wanted to move back to my home. I knew it would be a strain for my mother, moving from a house with a yard, back to my apartment that doesn't even have a balcony, but I was severely homesick.

So I packed up all my belongings and moved back to my place. As soon as we opened my door, I felt such as sigh of relief. Finally, I was able to return to resting in own bed.

About a month or so later, I had an appointment with my neurosurgeon. I actually went into Manhattan on my own for this appointment. I put on a headscarf to cover the incision before I left the house. Once I got to my doctor's office, he checked to see if my staples were ready to come out, and he affirmed that they were.

Get outta my head!

It didn't hurt to have them removed; it was more like a little pinch. Then he gave me some good news. He said that I could return to my normal routine, which included going back to work, exercising, and driving. Who would have thought, in less than 4 months after having brain surgery that I could go back to the things that I was previously doing. So then I put my headscarf back on, and headed home, with the biggest smile on my face.

Chapter Three
My cancer

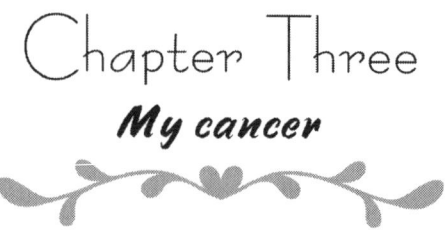

> "The best thing for you to do is to stop obsessing about cancer as something to fear! Flow with it, see it not as an intruder or grim reaper but see it as a friend that is helping you change your life and lifestyle."
> ~ Dr. Dennis Robinson ~

AFTER MY INITIAL surgery, my neurosurgeon had a talk with me about my tumor. He told me that it was cancerous. In hearing about the many people who have cancer, it never felt so real until my doctor told me that I had brain cancer.

First of all, I wondered what causes a tumor and cancer. There are common factors in cancer. It's a substance called telomerase, and all cancers have it. This is an enzyme essential in protecting DNA during cell replication; telomerase helps us all grow to adulthood. Then it shuts off. However, in cancer patients, the telomerase turns back on and causes uncontrollable cell growth resulting in cancer.

My doctor said my tumor was a Grade II Glioma (out of 4 grades) on my left frontal lobe of my brain. He told me that a Glioma is a general term used to describe any tumor that stems from the supportive tissue of the brain.

I asked him how serious my cancer was. He explained by telling me that tumors are graded from I to 4 depending on the severity. I thought to myself, ok, at least mine was in the lower half of the scale.

I then asked how long did I have the tumor in my head, but he said that there was really no way to pinpoint how long it was there. It's not like that information would have helped me anyway, but I was just curious. Maybe if I knew long it was there I could backtrack to that point in my life to see what was going on.

Going back to the grading of tumors, there are four tumor grades - I, II, III, and IV. The higher the grade, the more (malignant) or cancerous the tumor is. The grading helps the doctor to better understand the patient's condition and helps them to plan treatment.

Grade I: These are the least malignant tumors and are usually associated with long-term survival. They grow slowly and surgery alone may be an effective treatment for this grade.

Grade II: These tumors are slow-growing and look slightly abnormal under a microscope. Some can spread into nearby normal tissue and recur, sometimes as a higher grade tumor. This is the grade that I have.

Grade III: There is not always a big difference between grade II and grade III tumors. The cells of a grade III tumor are actively reproducing abnormal cells, which like grade II tumors can grow into nearby normal brain tissue. These tumors tend to recur, often as a grade IV.

Grade IV: These are the most malignant tumors. They reproduce rapidly, can have a bizarre appearance when viewed under the microscope, and easily grow into nearby normal brain tissue. These grade IV tumors form new blood vessels so they can maintain their rapid growth.

Brain tumors do not discriminate. Primary brain tumors (which is what I have), are those that begin in the brain and tend to stay in the brain, and they occur in people of all ages, but they are more frequent in children and older adults. Metastatic brain tumors on the other hand are those that begin as a cancer elsewhere in the body and spread to the brain. These are more common in adults than in children.

Treatments for brain tumors are individualized for each patient. It can depend on the patient's age, general health, as well as size, location, type, and grade of the tumor. In most cases, surgery, radiation and chemotherapy are the main types of treatment. Also, steroids are used to treat and prevent brain swelling. The placing of a ventriculoperitoneal shunt (VP shunt) is sometimes used. This is a tube that is placed into the fluid filled spaces of the brain. The other end of the tube is placed into the abdomen to drain excess fluid that can build up in the brain and cause an increase in brain pressure. Sometimes, more than one treatment might be necessary.

I was very fortunate that surgery and steroids were the only treatments required for my brain tumor. I only had to stay on steroids for about a month or two.

As for the residual piece of tumor still in my brain, it can cause seizures; therefore I am taking anti-convulsant medication. Also, I have to get regular MRI's to determine if there is any change in tumor size.

Get outta my head!

A malignant *brain tumor, which is what I have, is* rarely hereditary and does not frequently spread to *other* areas of the body, but they sometimes may recur after treatment.

While I was still in the hospital, one of the best gifts I received was a book from my college track friend Matthew Comas. It was a book called "Living with a Brain Tumor". That book gave me a lot of detail about my condition that I was unaware of.

I knew a little bit about the brain, but in this book I learned a lot more information. The brain and spinal cord together form the central nervous system. The CNS is the core of our existence. It controls our personality, thoughts, memory, intelligence, speech and understanding, emotions, senses, and basic body functions.

Another thing I learned from the book is how a tumor develops. It starts from one abnormal brain cell that grows and divides when it is not supposed to. Then five things happen to allow it to continue to grow. First, the abnormal cell learns to stimulate its own growth. Second, the tumor cells lose their tumor suppressor genes. Third, the tumor cells learn to spread by a process called invasion. Fourth, the tumor cells hide themselves from normal immune cells by becoming invisible. And then fifth, they form new blood vessels in order to increase their own nutrient supply and enhance their growth.

Though the exact cause of the start of tumors is unknown, there are some risk factors to take into consideration. These factors can be environmental, such as being exposed to certain chemicals; what you eat or don't eat; physical activity level; and lifestyle choices such as tobacco and alcohol use.

Some of the symptoms of a brain tumor include: headaches, vomiting, nausea, seizures, personality changes, irritability, sensory and motor loss, hearing loss, vision loss, fatigue, depression, and behavioral and cognitive (thinking) changes.

I also learned that the brain is comprised of several parts, each having their own functions.

There are the Temporal lobes, located at the sides of the brain, which process sound, understanding and producing speech, and involved with various aspects of memory. The Occiptal lobes are located at the lower back of the head, and helps in receiving and processing visual information, and also helps to perceive shapes and colors. The Parietal lobes, found behind the frontal lobes, aids in controlling sensation such as hot and cold. The Brain stem, located at the base of the brain, regulates involuntary functions such as breathing, heart rate, blood pressure, swallowing. The Cerebellum, at the back of the brain, controls balance, movement and coordination. My tumor is located in the left frontal lobe of my brain. I'll get more into that in a later chapter.

Once I got home from the hospital, I did the terrible thing of researching the life expectancy span of a person with brain cancer. But then I said to myself, it really doesn't matter what the internet or any doctors will say to me, it would only be their best guess.

Before I started to do my research, I recall developing a really deep connection with a television character in regards to cancer. It was October 24, 2010 and I was watching the Showtime series "The Big C" about a woman who has cancer. The main character, Cathy, reminded me of myself in that she reacted to her cancer in the same type of nonchalant manner in which I did. It wasn't until she was speaking to her doctor about how long she has to live, that I realized that I never spoke with my doctor about how long I have. Instead, I choose to just look it up on my own.

At first, I thought that unless some freak accident takes my life, I'll likely die from cancer related issues before old age sets in. But then I realized that the doctors can only give me a ball park time frame based on generalities and can't speak specifically about me. Whether I have 6 months, 6 years, or 60 years, I likely wouldn't do much different than what I would plan to do anyway. So if there's something I want to do, big or small, I should just do it, and not let cancer be the deciding factor.

Chapter Four
My life before cancer

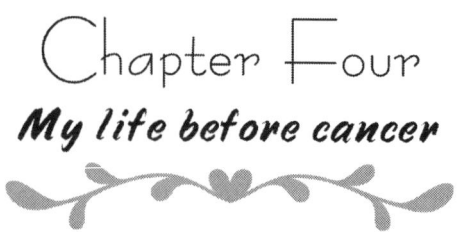

"Did you know that childhood is the only time in our lives when insanity is not only permitted to us, but expected?"
~ Louis de Bernières, Captain Corelli's Mandolin ~

I WAS BORN in Jamaica, West Indies to Alwyn and Ina Henry. I have 4 siblings, Garfield, Aqiyl, Toni and Krystal. My older brother and I were born in Jamaica, while the others were born in the United States. My older brother and I along with our parents stayed in Jamaica until I was 4 years old, and then we came to the U.S.

When I was young, we did a lot of moving around. We lived in Brooklyn when I first came to the states and this was where I started elementary school.

Then we moved from Brooklyn to Staten Island and then to Queens where I completed the bulk of my schooling. I currently stay in touch with quite a few friends from school, and many of them helped me through my bout with brain cancer. Some were able to visit me in the hospital, and others sent well wishes since they could not physically be there with me.

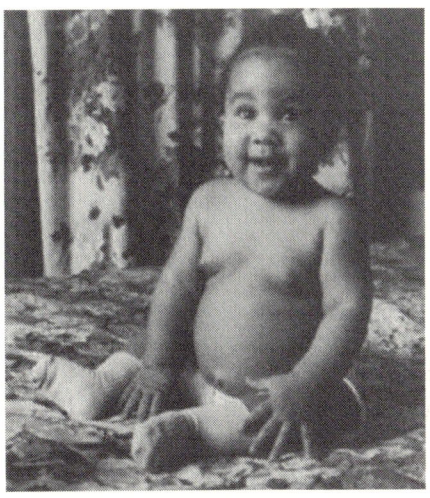

As a baby

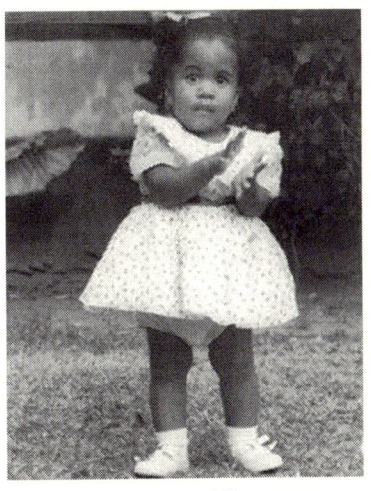

As a toddler

We grew up fairly close to our dad's parents, who lived in Manhattan. We would go to have dinner with them on most Sundays. I even lived with them for a while during the weekdays to cut down on my commute to work from Queens to Manhattan. After my grandfather retired, my grandparents moved to Florida and I would visit them, usually at Thanksgiving. My grandfather has since then passed away, on December 20, 2011.

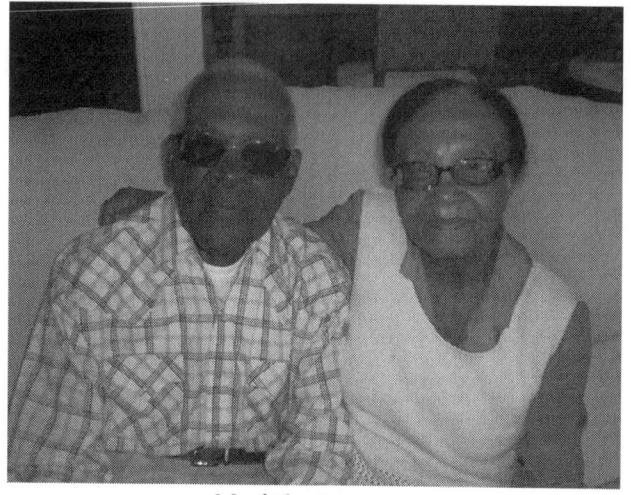

My father's parents

Again, I left Jamaica when I was four years old, and my mother's parents stayed behind. They both lived in Jamaica up to the time of my grandfather's death in 1981, so I did not see him past the age of four. My grandmother moved to the states when I was about 20 years old and she passed away when I was about 25 years of age.

Growing up as siblings, some of us had very contentious relationships at first, but what family doesn't. What brought us closer together as a family was when we all found out that I had brain cancer.

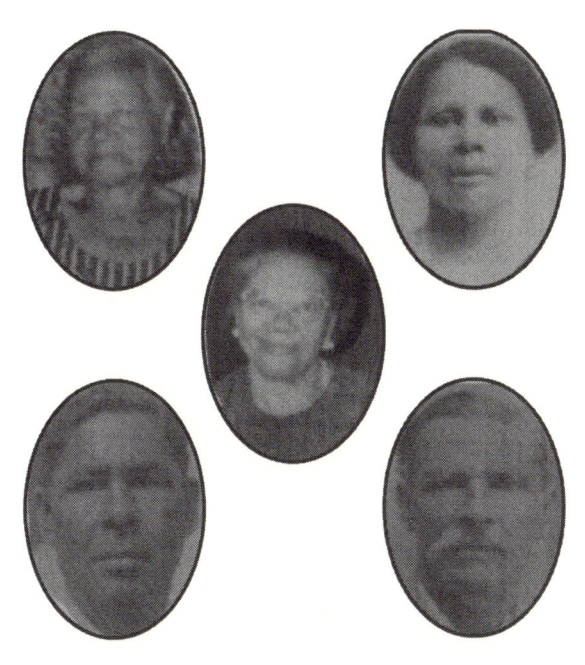

My mother's family

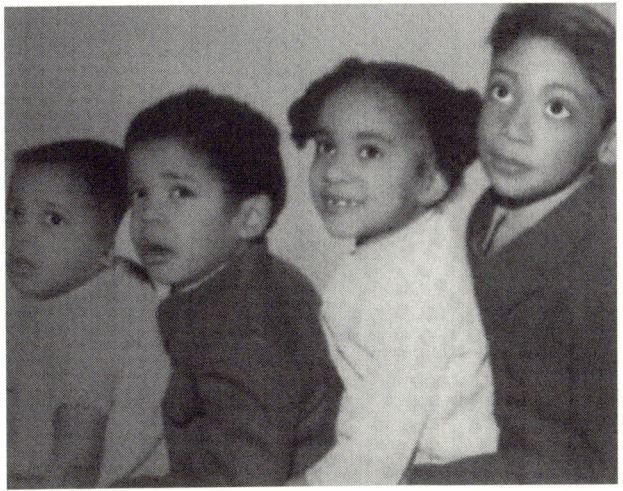

My sister Toni, my brother Aqiyl, me, my brother Garfield

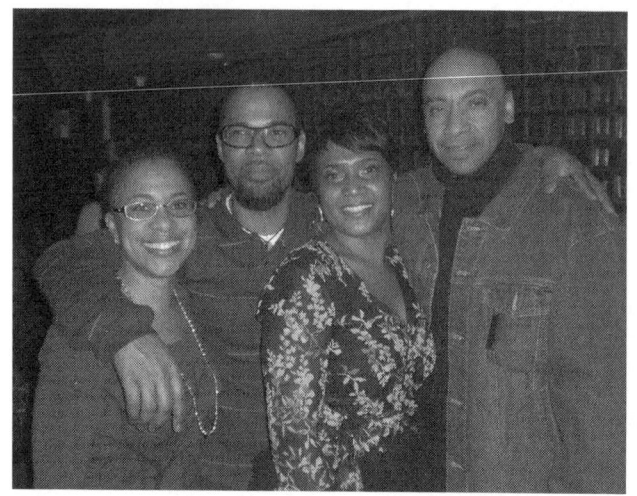

Me, my brother Aqiyl, my sister Toni, my brother Garfield

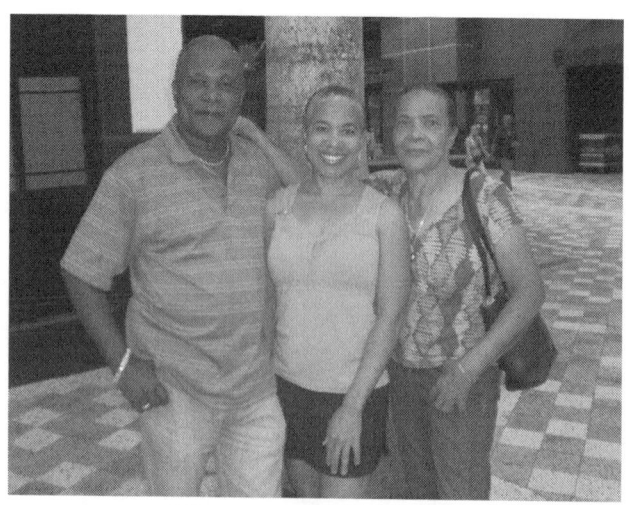

My parents and I in Florida

College Days

"Seek knowledge from the cradle to the grave."
~ Author unknown ~

Before I was diagnosed with brain cancer, I finished high school and immediately went to college. However, I did not finish out my first semester. I just felt totally unprepared, unlike my sister Toni who went to college straight out of high school and acquired her degree with no breaks in between.

Since I didn't finish out my first semester, my older brother Garfield put me in touch with a temporary agency where I got my first assignment as an accounting clerk at age 19, at Standard & Poor's, which is a rating agency.

Fast forward, I'm approximately in my upper 20's. Even though I didn't complete college right after high school, it was always a goal to eventually go back to school. So, I enrolled in York College in Jamaica, Queens.

For my freshman and sophomore years, I went to college part time majoring in Business Administration, while continuing to work full time. As part of the curriculum, I was required to take some classes that were not part of my actual major. My least favorite course was speech class. Some of my favorite classes were law and theatre. We also had to take a course which I enjoyed which was to take a class where we picked an alternate career path. I chose teaching as my back up career. We had to do actual field work, so I sat in on a teacher's class who I knew, which happened to be my sister Toni's class, and observed as she was teaching.

I eventually graduated from college with a degree in Business Administration with a 3.7 GPA, but my greatest honor was being selected CUNY (City University of New York) Scholar Athlete of the year, as part of being on the track team, which I'll get into later in this book.

It was my hope that this award would help to inspire others and show them that if you desire something badly enough that you can obtain it. You can work full time; attend college full time while being a full time athlete. My plate was quite full at this point, but I wanted this badly enough to go after it.

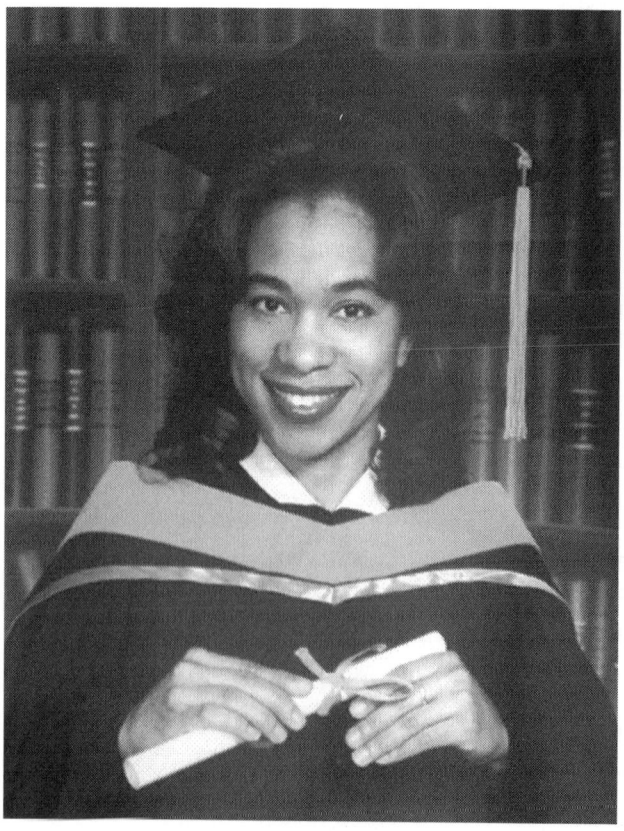

Graduation photo

My Career

"Choose a job you love, and you will never have to work a day in your life."
~ Confucius ~

During my 25+ years working at Standard & Poor's, I started out as an Accounting clerk, progressed to Secretary, Administrative Assistant, Research Analyst, Senior Research Analyst, Financial Analyst, Senior Financial Analyst, and then Manager/Financial Analysis.

Fast forward again. After my brain surgery, I returned to work about 4 months later, but only on a part time basis. I thought this was pretty quick for someone who just had brain surgery, but my neurosurgeon gave me the okay.

There was a new financial system in place when I returned to work. All the staff had 2 entire off site workdays to complete the training. My then supervisor stood over my shoulder and expected me to learn it in 15 minutes. But in light of just having brain surgery, I think I made the best of an awful situation.

Shortly after I returned to work, my supervisor quit the job. Then a co-worker, Joan, was moved into the supervisory role for our group. Joan was absolutely the best boss that anyone could ever ask for. She was patient and explained things in a manner conducive to understanding. She developed the group into a wonderful working atmosphere. I don't think anyone could ask for a better set of co-workers. We truly got along very well with each other, and I call them not just co-workers, but my friends.

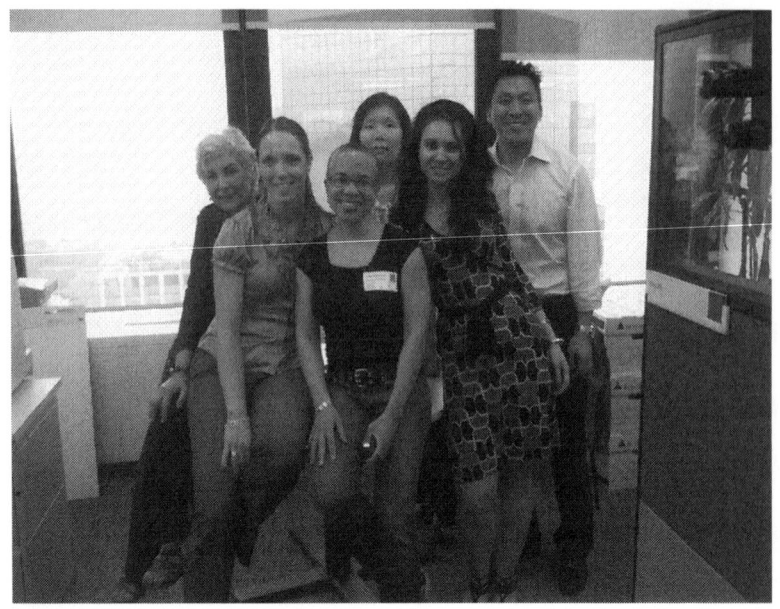

Co-workers

SPORTS

> *"Desire is the most important factor in the success of any athlete."*
> ~ Willie Shoemaker ~

As I speak about each sport, I will speak about how my seizures currently impact that activity, however, I won't get into the specific details of my seizures at this time.

When I was in high school, I joined the gymnastics team. That was the first sport that I participated in. One year, I qualified for the city championship on the floor exercise. Then one day during practice, I tore a ligament in my knee and had to have surgery.

I returned back to gymnastics while still in high school. However, I am no longer active in that sport, but I do enjoy watching it. Even if I wanted to participate in gymnastics at this point in my life, I doubt that my doctor would allow me to get involved with that sport again, due to my seizures.

Then when I was in my mid-20's I took to body building. I loved getting in shape and toning up. I even entered a body building competition. However, a few weeks before my 1st show, I injured my shoulder and could not participate. I've since then stopped trying to compete, however, I pin up pictures of bodybuilding women as my inspiration of the shape I'd like to get into. Again, my doctor doesn't want me to do any weight lifting without someone to assist me for fear of me having a seizure while lifting heavy equipment.

Then came my favorite sport which is running. I started track in my junior year and fell in love with it. In my senior year, we got a new coach, Mr. Pope. He had such a positive influence over me and I'll never forget it. I could not make regular practice times, but since he saw that I was dedicated, he extended practice to accommodate me. I appreciate all that he did for me and all the support he gave me in doing the thing I have such a great passion for.

I was very honored that a picture of me racing at a track meet graced the inside cover of our college yearbook. I did a series of races that landed me a spot to run at Madison Square Garden. I came in dead last, but just the privilege of running at the Garden was a magnificent honor. My favorite sport will likely always be running, both as a participant and an observer.

Even after graduating from college, my running days continued. As previously mentioned, I joined the running team at my company. I did fairly well, good enough for my score to count in almost all the races. Then I ran two half marathons, and the 2007 New York City Marathon.

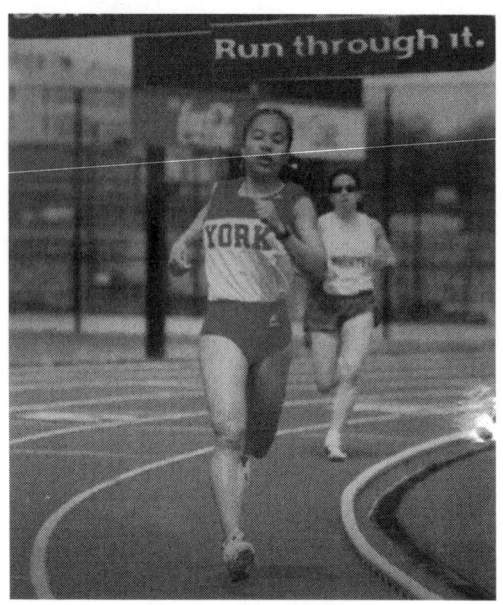

Track days

Currently, my running is on hiatus. I'm not allowed to run on a treadmill for if I have a seizure, I would go flying off and injure myself. Also, I can only run outdoors if I have a running partner, which I have yet to find one. Therefore, there will be no more running for me for the time being.

When I was in my early 40's, I stumbled upon yoga. That was one thing that I would have never thought I would like. But one day I was at the gym and friends kept telling me about how good the yoga class was. So I took it and loved it. This is an activity that I am still able to do even with my current illness.

Before going out of work on disability, I started to take boot camp classes. We had the most wonderful instructor. The class was only once a week, but it was awesome. A fellow gym buddy told me that she saw the improvement in my body since taking his class. That made my day. This type of intense activity level is definitely not something that my doctor would allow me to continue with at this point in time.

Friends

"It takes a long time to grow an old friend."
~ John Leonard ~

Over the course of my life, I've built a few wonderful, meaningful and lasting friendships. As I speak about each friend, I may speak on how they helped me to cope with my illness, but again, I'll get into more details on that in a later chapter.

When I was around 15 years old, my family used to take trips to Philadelphia to visit family. While I was there, I met my longest lasting friend, Mike Shannon. Mike and I continued to keep in touch writing letters to each other. His continued friendship has been a blessing to me through my battle dealing with cancer. Even though he could not be with me physically, he was always there in spirit and I knew I could reach out to him at a moment's whim.

Then I met my friend Marsha at a barbeque she was hosting at her home. We clicked and have been friends since then. She was there with me so many days and nights while I was in the hospital. She would even stay at my home with me on weekends.

I recall one particular night that she stayed over my home. During the early morning, she had gotten up to use the bathroom, and on her way out, she heard a banging from my bedroom. She came in to find me having a seizure and I had fallen over and my head was banging against my nightstand.

She pulled me back to the middle of my bed and called 911. The paramedics took me to the hospital and Marsha met me there. – They took blood work, kept an eye on me, and released me the same day.

Then I met another friend, Laverne. We met competing against each other at track meets. She beat me all except one time. That was the time that I was sick from a cold and had taken so much medication. I joked with Laverne that it was the cold medications that made me run faster!

I recall one day I was at Laverne's home, and before she would leave for work, she was going to drive me part of the way back home, and then I would take public transportation the rest of the way. As we were about to leave her home, I slid to the floor and had a seizure. Then I had another, and another. After about the 5th seizure, her friend called 911 and they took me to the hospital. By the end of that day, I probably had about 15 seizures. This time, they kept me in the hospital for about a week and ran various tests, then released me once the seizures were under control.

When I was about 20 years old, I met Genny at the place where we both worked. She has since then moved on to another job, but while we were employed at this job, we quickly became very good friends.

I was a bridesmaid at her wedding and she was maid of honor at mine. We were there for each other throughout our respective marriages and for our divorces as well. For a brief period in time, we lost contact, but then we hooked back up together and it was as if no time had elapsed during our separation.

I recall the day of Genny's college graduation. I had spent the night at her home the day before. As we're getting dressed and preparing to leave, I had about 2 seizures. They didn't last long, and I was so glad that it was only 2, but I was afraid that my seizures would interfere with her graduation day, but luckily they did not. She just kept an eye on me as we drove to her graduation. I think she told her family what happened, that way they too would keep an eye on me.

Knowing that I could no longer drive due to my seizures, Genny would take time off from work to take me to doctor's appointments. During her family gatherings, she would pick me up and drop me back home, just so that I could attend the functions. This meant an awful lot of out of the way driving on her part, but that's the kind of friend she is.

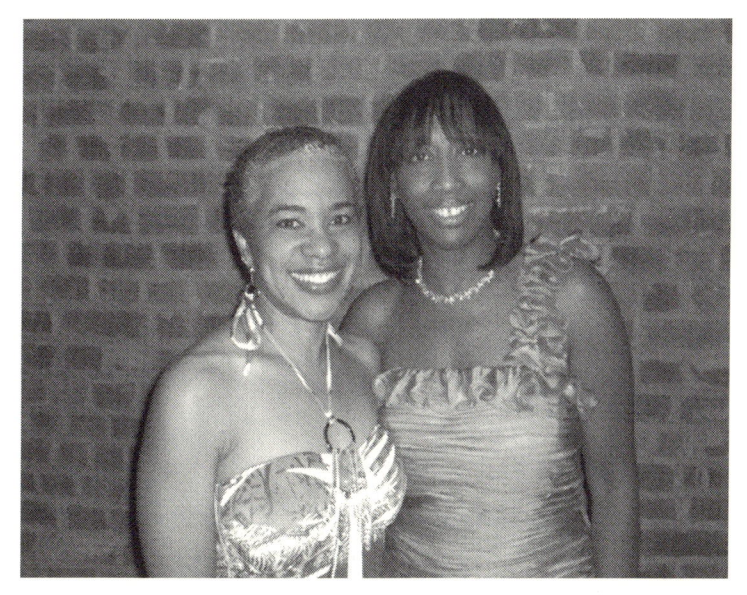

Me and Genny

Chapter Five
Cancer can hit anyone

"At any given moment, cancer can hit you. So instead of denying it, I've owned my cancer. Therefore, I decided to give my cancer colors. What color is my cancer? It's the colors of a rainbow. That puts me in a cheerful, colorful mood.

"Some might ask 'Wouldn't it be better if you never had a tumor and cancer to begin with?' But I see the good in things. I have a malignant tumor, and I can't do anything about it now. I have a much better outlook on life since finding this out. It has given me the platform to write about it, and to lend support, encourage and uplift others in need of comfort. So I accept my cancer, embrace it, and give it nice bright colors."
~ Collette A. Henry ~

I HAD AN average childhood and young adulthood. I went to college, engaged in sports, and had my career and my share of friendships. I didn't do any of the things associated with deliberately bringing about cancer.

I didn't smoke. I've only had desk jobs, so I doubt I was exposed to chemicals, hazardous materials or radiation. I did not overexpose myself to sunlight, never got into a tanning bed, and never had a virus or bacteria that required medical attention.

I took precaution as far as certain risk factors. I always maintained a healthy body weight for my age and height. I was into physical activity starting with high school. I don't know if I've had the healthiest of diets, however whenever I went for annual checkups, I always received a good report.

According to National Cancer Institute, for my particular type of cancer, as of 2012, it was estimated that 22,910 men and women (12,630 men and 10,280 women) would be diagnosed with cancer of the brain and other nervous systems.

According to WebMd, Livestrong, Centers for Disease Control, and the Mayo Clinic, more than one million people in the United States gets cancer each year. So, to "reduce" the risk of cancer, these organizations say:

Do not smoke. Using any type of tobacco puts you in danger with cancer. Smoking has been linked to various types of cancer, including cancer of the lung, bladder, cervix and kidney. Also, chewing tobacco has been linked to cancer of the oral cavity and pancreas. Even if you don't use tobacco, exposure to secondhand smoke might increase your risk of lung cancer. Combined, lung cancer kills more women and men in the U.S. than any other cancer.

Watch your diet. Limit consumption of calorie-dense foods, particularly processed foods high in added sugar, low in fiber or high in fat. Eat plenty of fruits and vegetables, and plant sources such as whole grains and beans. Limit consumption of red meats such as beef, pork, lamb, and avoid processed meat. Limit consumption of salty foods and foods processed with sodium.

Be as lean as possible without becoming underweight. Maintaining a healthy weight might lower risk of certain types of cancer, including breast, prostate, lung, colon and kidney cancer. Many people probably know that carrying too much weight around isn't good for your heart, but it's also a major risk factor for cancer as well. Obesity is the cause behind approximately 15% of cancer deaths.

Work out. Physical activity counts as well in lowering certain types of cancer, like breast and colon cancer. All forms of physical activity help to prevent many forms of cancer. You may not get the six-pack abs with 30 minutes of moderate exercise every day, but a number of studies have found evidence that just this much physical activity can cut your risk of many common cancers by 30% to 50%.

Avoid midday sun; use sunscreen; avoid tanning beds and sunlamps.

Get immunized. Hepatitis B can increase the risk of developing liver cancer.

Practice safe sex. Use a condom if you have sex. If you have unprotected sex, the more sexual partners you have, the more likely you are to contract a sexually transmitted disease or sexual virus/infection. People who have HIV or AIDS have a higher risk of cancer of the anus, liver and lung. And the Human Papilloma virus (HPV) is most often associated with cervical cancer, but it might also increase the risk of cancer of the anus, penis, throat, vulva and vagina.

Don't share needles. Sharing needles with an infected drug user can lead to HIV, as well as hepatitis B and hepatitis C, which can increase the risk of liver cancer

Shake off stress. There's no convincing evidence that, by itself, stress is an independent risk factor for cancer. But what it can do to you is engage you in unhealthy behavior in an effort to cope with stress. If you're overeating, drinking, or smoking to self-medicate your stress away, those activities all raise your cancer risk. So instead, find healthy ways of coping with stress, like exercise (which helps to reduce you chance of getting cancer), meditation, and journaling.

Get regular medical care. Regular self-exams and screenings for various types of cancers, such as cancer of the skin, colon, prostate, cervix and breast, can increase your chances of discovering cancer early, when treatment is most likely to be successful. Mammograms and prostate-specific antigen (PSA) testing, catch cancer at a very early stage, when it may be more treatable. Other tests, like Pap tests and colonoscopies, can help detect precancerous cells that, if left untreated, can turn into cervical cancer or colon cancer.

Look into your roots. Learn about your family health history in detail. This can create a strategy for catching cancer risk early.

According to Center for Disease control (CDC), the 10 most commonly diagnosed cancers among "men" in the United States include:

1) Prostate: symptoms include a need to urinate frequently; difficulty starting urination; weak or interrupted flow of urine; painful or burning urination, difficulty in getting an erection, painful ejaculation, blood in urine or semen, frequent pain or stiffness in the lower back, hips, or upper thighs.

For 2012, it was estimated that 241,740 men would be diagnosed with prostate cancer.

2) Lung: symptoms include chronic cough, shortness of breath, chronic mucus production, wheezing, coughing up blood, chronic chest pain.

3) Colon and rectum: symptoms include stomach pain, bloody stools or dark stools, change in bowel habits, constant tiredness or fatigue and rarely unexplained weight loss.

4) Bladder: symptoms include blood or blood clots in the urine, pain during urination, urinating small amounts frequently, frequent urinary tract infections, pain in the lower back around the kidney, swelling in the lower legs, a growth in pelvis near the bladder.

5) Melanomas of the skin: symptoms include a small lump (spot or mole) that is shiny, waxy, pale in color, and smooth in texture; a red lump (spot or mole) that is firm; a sore or spot that bleed or becomes crusty (also look for sores that don't heal); rough and scaly patches on the skin; flat scaly areas of the skin that are red or brown.

6) Non-Hodgkin lymphoma: symptoms include night sweats (even though room temperature is not too hot), fever and chills that come and go; itching, swollen lymph nodes in neck, underarms, and groin, weight loss, coughing or shortness of breath, abdominal pain or swelling which may lead to a loss of appetite, constipation, nausea and vomiting.

7) Kidney: symptoms include blood in your urine, a lump in your side of abdomen, loss of appetite, pain in your side that doesn't go away, weight loss for no reason, fever that lasts for weeks and isn't caused by a cold or other infection, extreme fatigue, anemia, swelling in your ankles of legs.

8) Mouth and throat: symptoms include a painless lump on the lip, in the mouth, or in the throat, a sore on the lip or include the mouth that does not heal, a painless white or red patch on the gums, tongue, or lining of the mouth; unexplained pain, bleeding, or numbness inside the mouth; a sore throat that does not go away; pain or difficulty with chewing or swallowing; swelling of the jaw, hoarseness or other change in the voice.

9) Leukemias: symptoms include fever or chills;, persistent fatigue or weakness, frequent infections, losing weight without trying, swollen lymph nodes, easy bleeding or bruising, tiny red spots on your skin, excessive sweating especially at night, bone pain or tenderness.

10) Pancreas: symptoms include upper abdominal pain that may radiate to your back, yellowing of your skin and the whites of your eyes, loss of appetite, weight loss, depression, blood clots.

The 10 most commonly diagnosed cancers among "women" in the United States include:

Breast: symptoms include a lump or thickening in the breast or underarm area that feels different from the surrounding tissue; abnormal or bloody discharge from the nipple; change in the size or shape of the breast, inverted nipple; any abnormal change in the skin over the breast or the nipple such as dimpling, redness, pitting (like the skin of an orange), peeling or flaking of the nipple or breast skin. Breast self-exams and mammography can help early detection of breast cancer when it is most treatable.

For 2012, it was estimated that 226,870 women would be diagnosed with breast cancer.

Lung: symptoms include chronic cough, shortness of breath, chronic mucus production, wheezing, coughing up blood, chronic chest pain.

Colon and rectum: symptoms include stomach pain, bloody stools or dark stools, change in bowel habits, constant tiredness or fatigue and rarely unexplained weight loss.

Uterus: symptoms include abnormal vaginal bleeding, spotting or discharge, pain or difficulty when empting the bladder, pain during sex, pain in the pelvic area.

Thyroid: symptoms include a lump or swelling in neck, pain in our neck and sometimes in your ears, trouble swallowing, trouble breathing or constant wheezing, a hoarse throat, frequent cough not related to a cold. Some people may not have any symptoms. Their doctors may find a lump or nodule in the neck during a routine physical exam.

Non-Hodgkin lymphoma: symptoms include night sweats (even though room temperature is not too hot), fever and chills that come and go, itching, swollen lymph nodes in neck, underarms, and groin; weight loss, coughing or shortness of breath, abdominal pain or swelling which may lead to a loss of appetite, constipation, nausea and vomiting.

Melanomas of the skin: symptoms include a small lump (spot or mole) that is shiny, waxy, pale in color, and smooth in texture; a red lump (spot or mole) that is firm, a sore or spot that bleed or becomes crusty (also look for sores that don't heal), rough and scaly patches on the skin, flat scaly areas of the skin that are red or brown.

Ovarian: symptoms include vaginal bleeding or discharge from your vagina that is not normal for you, pain in the pelvic or abdominal area (below your stomach and between your hip bone), back pain, bloating, feeling full quickly while eating, a change in bathroom habits such as having to pass urine very badly or very often, constipation or diarrhea.

Kidney: symptoms include blood in your urine, a lump in your side of abdomen, loss of appetite, pain in your side that doesn't go away, weight loss for no reason, fever that lasts for weeks and isn't caused by a cold or other infection; extreme fatigue, anemia, swelling in your ankles of legs.

Pancreas: symptoms include upper abdominal pain that may radiate to your back, yellowing of your skin and the whites of your eyes, loss of appetite, weight loss, depression, blood clots.

Chapter Six
Fallout and treatments

"The only thing that should surprise us is that there are still some things that can surprise us."
~ Francois de La Rochefoucauld ~

AS MENTIONED IN Chapter 1, finding out that I had a tumor and cancer all started with me having a seizure. When the brain is functioning properly, it sends a sort of energy to different parts of itself. But as for me, my brain cells kept sending energy in an abnormal manner. This caused me to have my first seizure. As time went on, I had others.

Since this had become a part of my life, I started to look into seizures. Many people have a misconception that you should place something in the mouth of someone having a seizure. But that's not the case, and you could just cause further injury to the person if you do that. What you should do is place something soft under their head. I'm sure on the occasion of my initial seizure, there wasn't time to do this, since I fell and hit the pavement. You should then loosen tight clothing, such as anything close to their neck, like a tie. But since I was partaking in a race, I didn't have on any restrictive clothing.

You should also try not to restrain the person's movements during their seizure unless there are objects around that they can harm themselves with. If possible, just move those objects away. Also, try to turn the person on their side to open the airway to allow secretions to drain from their mouth. Loss of bladder control could occur, but I'm glad that wasn't the case for me.

So, after I was taken to the hospital, I had my brain surgery, which was all that was required. I'm fortunate that I didn't have to undergo radiation or chemotherapy treatment for the residual tumor still in my brain. But here's a little background on those treatments.

RADIATION

More than half of all cancer patients receive some type of radiation therapy, which uses much more powerful x-ray energy than is used to take a simple x-ray. The goal of radiation is to stop cancer cells from multiplying while at the same time sparing as much healthy tissue as possible.

Radiation therapy is needed in various situations such as:

Before surgery to try to shrink the tumor

During surgery to aim large doses directly at a tumor

After surgery to help stop the growth of any remaining cancer cells

To decrease pressure and pain during cancers that unfortunately can't be cured.

Radiation side effects can include fatigue as well as sunburn-like burns to the skin where the radiation beam was focused.

Chemotherapy

Chemotherapy uses drugs, or chemicals, to kill cells that are rapidly dividing. These cells include both cancer cells and healthy cells. Most chemotherapy is given as a combination of drugs that work together to kill as many cancer cells as possible.

Chemotherapy works by stopping or slowing the growth of cancer cells. But it can also harm healthy cells that divide quickly.

Chemotherapy may be given in many ways:

Injection. The chemotherapy is given by a shot in a muscle in your arm, thigh, or hip or right under the skin in the fatty part of your arm, leg, or belly.

Intra-arterial (IA). The chemotherapy goes directly into the artery that is feeding the cancer.

Intraperitoneal (IP). The chemotherapy goes directly into the peritoneal cavity (the area that contains organs such as your intestines, stomach, liver, and ovaries).

Intravenous (IV). The chemotherapy goes directly into a vein.

Topically. The chemotherapy comes in a cream that you rub onto your skin.

Orally. The chemotherapy comes in pills, capsules, or liquids that you swallow.

Damage to healthy cells may cause side effects. Often, these side effects get better or go away after chemotherapy is over.

Some side effects include:

One of the most serious potential side effects is a low count of white blood cells. White blood cells help your body fight infection by protecting against foreign invaders such as bacteria and viruses.

Hair loss, fatigue, nausea. Ginger can be used to try to offset the nausea. The truth is, chemotherapy affects everyone differently. And many of the negative effects can be controlled through medications.

Another side effect is anemia, which is low red blood cell count.

Now that I have a residual piece of the tumor in my brain, it has caused me to have more seizures, and therefore I have to take anticonvulsant medication.

Seizures are not a disease in themselves. Instead, they are a symptom of many different disorders that can affect the brain. Most seizures last only a minute or two, although confusion afterwards may last longer.

Here's a little more background on different types of seizures I have and ways my doctors are helping to monitor them:

Epileptic seizures are convulsions accompanies by impaired consciousness (though not necessarily a total loss of consciousness.)

Non elliptic seizures (or PNES - Psychogenic non epileptic seizure) are superficial events resembling an epileptic seizure, but without the characteristic of electrical discharges. PNES are regarded as psychological in origin. The most conclusive test to distinguish epilepsy from PNES is long term video-EEG monitoring (Electroencephalography.)

EEG-video is used for patients who continue to have frequent seizures despite being on antiepileptic drugs (which was my case.) An EEG is the recording of electrical activity along the scalp.

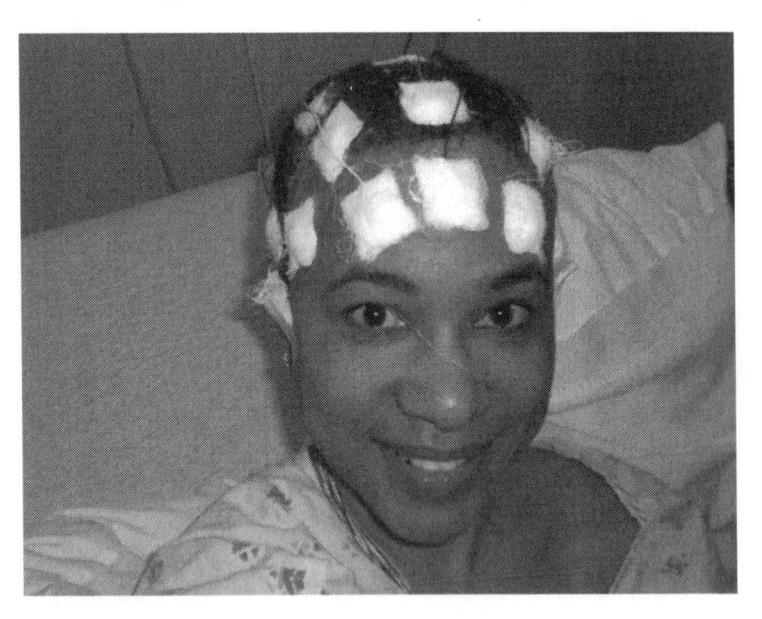

My video EEG monitoring

The purpose of this type of monitoring is to answer the following questions:
Are the episodes epileptic seizure?
If not, what are they?

It took several EEG tests to reveal that I have both epileptic seizures and PINES. The latter have made up the bulk of my 200 plus seizures since May of 2009. Most PNES patients are women, with the onset in the late teen to early twenties being typical; however for me it was later in life. PNES patients often have a history of multiple vague unexplained medical problems and have a psychiatric condition such as major depression or anxiety disorder.

Not all seizures cause you to lose consciousness. My 1st seizure from returning back to work was back in November 2009. I was sitting at my desk with a co-worker when all of a sudden I put my hands on my head and told her that I wasn't feeling well. My head started to deviate violently to my right side and I started to scream at the top of my lungs, as though I was in physical pain, even though I wasn't. Then my body started jerking. I was fully aware of what was happening.

I could hear everything around me, but my eyes were closed. I heard my manager tell our assistant to call for an ambulance. My seizure was over before the EMT personnel arrived. They asked me a series of questions to see if I was lucid, and then took me to the hospital.

I think the most frustrating thing about having a seizure is coming to the full realization that during those moments, I have lost control over my mind and body. I always used to think I was stronger than that, and it's quite a humbling thing to realize that not everything is in my control.

I've often been asked to describe what it feels like to be in the midst of a seizure. During a seizure where I don't lose consciousness, I describe it as imagining the movies "Nightmare on Elm Street" crossed with "Misery." That's what my head feels like when I have a seizure. It's like my mind is trapped in a horror movie that I can't wake up from, and I feel totally paralyzed to do anything to free myself from it. During a seizure that I do lose consciousness, the last thing I'm aware of is that my head starts to violently jerk to my right side like a scene out of "The Exorcist."

Then in May of 2010, the 1st year anniversary of being diagnosed with brain cancer, I ended back up in the hospital again due to seizures. I was in the hospital this time for about a week, where I had 35 seizures during this time period. Once released, I was out of work again from May 2010 and did not return back until August 2010.

My return to work after August was very brief. I kept having more seizures to the point where I had to go out of work on long term disability starting in October 2010, and I am currently still out on disability due to my seizures.

As for my epileptic seizures, my neurologist has me on just one anticonvulsant medication. It took a while before we got to a medication that worked well for me. I started out on Keppra which was doing fine for about 5 months. But then I began to have more seizures. So my medication was increased. I still continued to have seizures, so my medication was increased further to the point where I developed a rash. Then my doctor changed my medication to my current one, Lamictal, which is working well with no side effects.

For my psychogenic seizures (which make up the bulk of my seizures), I was required to seek psychiatric help. My psychiatrist diagnosed me with an anxiety disorder. I am currently taking two different medications under her care, but the goal is to wean me down to just one medication.

I am also under the care of a psychologist for regular therapy sessions to determine the cause of my anxiety. She feels that my brain had "subconsciously" learned to have seizures when I'm stressed. She compares it to a pair of pantyhose. After the pantyhose have been worn, after you wash them, they still retain the shape of your foot. My brain has subconsciously retained the ability to have seizures when I'm anxious; stressed or when my body is out of balance.

As for the tumor, I get brain MRI's twice a year to see if the tumor has changed in size. Since May of 2009, it has not changed.

While many people just have just a few doctors, I now have a team of doctors that include my neurosurgeon, neurologist (who I see every 3 months), oncologist (who I see twice a year), a psychiatrist and a psychologist who I see both on a monthly basis.

As far as life changes, this has impacted my life in the area that I like the most - working out. When I first found out from my neurologist that I could start to run again, he said only if I wear a helmet and I was with someone. So I purchased a helmet, but I didn't go running out of sheer embarrassment. Then after time passed he said I could run helmet free, still provided that someone was with me. So as for now, I can basically only do things such as yoga and pilates.

Chapter Seven
Who am I?

"There used to be a real me, but I had it surgically removed."
~ Peter Sellers ~

SINCE HAVING BRAIN surgery, I'm left wondering, who is the real Collette? Was pre-surgery with the tumor the real me, or is post-surgery with a piece of tumor still intact the real one, or is it a combination of both? Will I be the real Collette if only the entire tumor could have been removed?

As previously stated, my tumor is in my frontal lobe, which among other things, controls memory.

For as long back as I can recall, I've always had memory problems. (That is such an oxymoron.) I don't recall growing up in Jamaica at all. I was only 4 years old when I left, but I have family members who can recall that early stage of their childhood.

I don't remember living in Staten Island either, and that was when I was a pre-teen, so I should have some memories of that period in my life.

My memory problems are the reverse of my sister Toni, who remembers quite a lot of details from when we were children. She was always puzzled that I could not remember details of my own life, even things that happened in my twenties.

I wonder if I had the tumor at this point in time, and if it was just starting to grow and beginning to wreak havoc in my brain, thus causing my memory problems. I guess I'll never know.

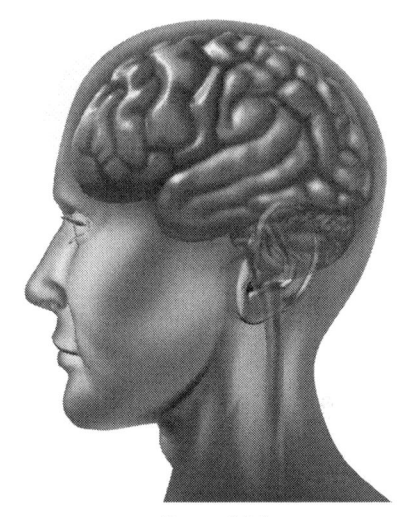

Frontal lobe

As stated, my residual tumor is in my frontal lobe which is located behind the forehead. These lobes serve many functions, basically including the "essence" of our humanity.

They control impulse decisions. I would say that I have made quite a lot of bad decisions in my life, hurting many people based on my impulsive nature. I think my personal relationships are a good reflection of this.

For example, I was easily able to just get up and walk away from a relationship. It wasn't as though we were having problems that were slowly coming to a head. Instead, one day I just woke up and felt like I just didn't want to be with that person anymore.

I'm very impetuous when it comes to entering a relationship in the first place. I don't give it time for us to develop a friendship, just jumped right into "we are in a (romantic) relationship".

When I was in my very early 20's, I met a guy and it didn't take long before I moved in with him. This was one of the more impulsive things that I had done.

The frontal lobes also controls decision making. I was engaged three times. During one of these engagements, I think the long term outcome would have been that one of us would be dead and the other person in prison. I wonder if pre-tumor, Collette would have even gotten involved with someone of that nature that could have possibly ended in such a tragic way.

Also, I used to be married. It didn't last long, only 3 years. He is a very good man, who deserved better than I treated him. We had previously made 2-3 attempts at a relationship, and then decided to get married. I don't generally go back to a relationship once it has ended, but I do wonder what changed in this situation. Could my tumor have had some affect?

Also, I wonder if my decision to start to work right out of high school was tumor related. It seemed the best option at the time, but I wonder how different my life would have been if I decided to not only go to college right after high school, but to move far away from home, like my sister did.

This is not an attempt to blame all my prior actions on my tumor, I'm just curious about what if it was the tumor all along influencing my decisions.

These frontal lobes also control selective attention, and maybe that's why I sometimes have a hard time focusing on one project at a time.

They also control our sexual behavior, judgment and emotions relating to sympathy. It also influences functions relating to understanding humor, and ability to recognize sarcasm and irony. Other functions include the ability to perform a multi-step task like making a sandwich.

The frontal lobe also controls the ability to solve problems and the ability to express language correctly. They also manage movement, initiation, planning, and organizing.

Injury to the frontal lobes after surgery may affect:

Emotions

Impulse control: I've been told that I've become more impulsive

Language: I've noticed that I sometimes have a hard time putting my thoughts into words

Memory: I feel as though my memory has deteriorated

Social behavior

Sexual behavior

In a nutshell, our personalities are controlled by the frontal lobes. Considering this, I wonder how different my personality would have been if I did not have a brain tumor. And since I still have a piece of the tumor in my brain, I wonder if my personality would change even further if it were to be removed.

Chapter Eight
Life goes on

"Throughout these last few years, with my 2 surgeries, trips to the lab, tests, and the plethora of doctors I've seen, I could have a pity party and whine, but my condition has given more medical students an opportunity to learn their craft, which I find pretty darn cool. There is always a bright side to everything."
~ Inspired by my friend Elizabeth A. Potter ~

NOW ON TO some of the things that I've been up to since my last disability stint that started in October 2010.

In my spare time, I developed some hobbies. Backtrack to when I was in my early twenties; I met a friend Gisela Cody. She showed me how to sew and crochet. The sewing I gave up, I just alter clothes now. However, I still crochet, mainly scarves and baby blankets.

Also, while out of work, I decided to get a puppy, who I named CJ. Her favorite thing to do was to bite the staples out of cable wires that I had along the floor. She was quite a handful.

My psychiatrist cautioned me on getting a full night of sleep. However, CJ would not allow for that. At nighttime, she wouldn't let me sleep because she kept making constant noise. I was starting to get roughly 2 hours of consecutive sleep each night.

Then I thought about C.J. and what would happen to her once I returned to work and was out of the house for at least 12 hours a day, sometimes even longer. She'd be alone all that time, with no one to even take her out for a walk. So that, coupled with my lack of sleep, I decided to give her up for adoption.

So now, what to do? I started to hang out with my friend Ty from theatre class in college. He was my movie and dinner buddy. Ty and I are also both in the same Facebook Fitness Forum Group, where we got into juicing for health purposes. Since I couldn't drive, he would go into Brooklyn to pick up the juices from a mutual friend, and drive back to Long Island to deliver them to me. I don't think he truly knows just how much I appreciated his efforts.

Also, during my disability periods, I wrote two articles for Harlem World Online Magazine. The main theme was cancer, but my articles spread into a lot of areas of my life. It covered physical pain, my brain infection, my seizures, my lack of sleep, the outpouring of concern, the healthcare system, and how I'm moving forward.

For my 1st article, I received a lot of positive feedback, mostly people encouraging me to keep up with my positive spirit and asking me to continue to write. Others said that by me writing about my journey it has helped them to put their lives in perspective and now they don't worry so much about the small stuff.

Then, sometime around May or June of 2012, I turned to blogging as another outlet of sharing my journey with others. It was fascinating not just writing, but reading other people's blogs.

While some people felt that my stories helped them, I found that some of the other bloggers stories helped me. It further helped me to realize how fortunate I was in that I'm not suffering through daily pain like they are. I didn't have to go through radiation treatment or chemotherapy and suffer some of the awful side effects that they did.

Also, my first informal speaking engagement came at a gathering where I went with my friend Genny. There was a band scheduled to play, but before they took stage, the microphone was open to the public. I went up on the stage and said "Hi, my name is Collette and I'm a brain cancer survivor." I think that was the first time I ever said those words out loud. I gave a brief speech and it felt really good. Luckily, this time, my fear from speech class did not come back to haunt me.

Aside from my articles, my blog, and my informal speaking engagement, I've done a couple of interviews. One day, a friend of mine who knows that I have cancer reached out to me to ask for my help. Her son had a class project to do where he had to interview someone with an illness, and I agreed to it. He called me and we had a conversation over the phone - he asked a slew of questions, such as when I was diagnosed to how I am dealing with it now. He earned a 93 and I am happy to have helped him achieve such a good grade!

In June 2012, I was approached to do a radio show interview. I said yes, but then I had flashbacks to my speech class and how nervous I was at public speaking. Even though this would be a radio broadcast, I still associated it as being the same as giving a speech in my class.

The show was set for June 23rd. About 3 weeks before the interview, the woman hosting the show called me and we had a very casual conversation over the phone where I told her my story.

She said that was exactly how she wanted the show to go. It was not to be scripted, but instead free flowing as though I was having a conversation with the audience. Then the day before the show, I had to set 2 alarm clocks to ensure that I got up on time. With an hour left before show time, I was in a panic.

I called in 15 minutes ahead of time so that they could do a sound check. The host started to speak to me, in a very calm manner, so now I was starting to feel at ease. Then show time!

She introduced herself to the audience and chatted with them for about two minutes, and then she introduced me to them. I immediately felt at ease. I just spoke as suggested, as though I was having a conversation with a friend. I didn't rush myself. I just went along at a nice, even pace. Once the half hour radio show was over, the host said that I did just fine.

Also, while out of work, I created a Facebook page called *"Collette Henry Brain Cancer Awareness"*. I use this tool as a place where I post inspiration, motivational and informational items regarding not just brain cancer, but cancer in general.

Through this site, I've come to learn about many people who also have varying types of cancer and other illnesses, and if I was able to be a source of comfort for anyone of them through my posts, then I felt that I succeeded at something.

I used this Facebook page as a springboard for my next project, a Facebook group called *"Collette's Cancer Support Group."* This is where those who have or had cancer and also for their caregivers to come together to share their stories. Right now, it's a small group, but my hope is that it grows further and many more stories are shared, and that many more words of encouragement can be passed on from one to another.

And now, with writing this book, I have established my own publishing company, Ettelloc Publishing, a play on words, which is my name spelled backwards.

So, what's life like for me now, since finding out about my tumor, cancer, and seizures?

As for the cancer, it's still only stage two out of four. As far my tumor, as mentioned; I just get MRI's every 6 months to see if the tumor is growing back or not. Since May 2009 to date, my tumor has remained unchanged in size.

However, of late, in regards to getting the MRI's, I've developed an allergic reaction to the dye that is used in the procedure. When getting a brain MRI, they put me in the machine for about 20 minutes. Then they take me out and inject a dye intravenously which is used to enhance the brain images. There was an occasion where as soon as they gave me the dye, within one minute my entire body started to itch and turn red.

They had to pull me out and immediately give me Benadryl. So now, as a precaution, I have to take a Benadryl before the dye is injected to try to counter my allergic reaction. But even with the Benadryl, I still get the itching and redness, but it would be worse without the pill.

With having cancer, one thing that I'm surprised about is that I thought it would have compromised my immune system and that I would be prone to getting sick more often. But that was not the case. One day I thought I felt the "inkling" of a cold coming on, so I went into my medicine cabinet to look for cold medicine. Lo and behold, everything had expired 2009, the year of my surgery.

At first I was so upset, but then a friend pointed out, hey that means you haven't caught a cold in 3 years! So now, I don't even bother with medications, if I get the inkling again, I just drink warm water with lemon or some other citrus and I feel better almost immediately.

As far as my seizures are concerned, I am still taking one medication prescribed from my neurologist and two from my psychiatrist, but again her goal is to wean me from two down to just one. I am also still seeing my psychologist to determine the root of my anxiety. She sometimes feels that I might also be in the beginning stages of depression. I don't feel depressed, but I guess there are patterns in my behavior or mood that she picks up on that I don't notice. We haven't come to a source of my anxiety but have uncovered other things; like that I might have a fear of relationship commitment. It's amazing the things you uncover in therapy, but I won't go into the itty bitty details.

Again, my psychiatrist has cautioned me on getting enough sleep. I've tried so many things. I wear earplugs. She put me on Valium, that didn't work. I went to a hypnotist, that didn't work. I tried Valerian Root and melatonin as recommended by my doctor, those didn't work. I have just about resigned myself to thinking that I just won't be able to get more than 3-4 hours of consistent sleep.

So, what else has been going on? Well, my sense of independence has changed. I've been very self-sufficient for such a long time, yet now I have learned to depend on others, which took a lot of adjusting to do on my part. I have not driven since November 2009 due to the seizures, and I actually gave my car to my ex-husband. Luckily most places that I need to go to are within walking distance, especially the grocery store.

However, until I got accustomed to going places on my own, my sister Toni, who lives a few towns from me, would often drive to pick me up and run errands with me. On many occasions when I had a seizure and was hospitalized, she was the one who would pick me up from the hospital to bring me home.

I recall one day I walked to the post office and when I left I had a seizure. I later told my sister about it. She lightly scolded me for not asking her to call her when I needed to go somewhere. It's quite amusing having your younger sister admonish you. She still drives me to places too far for me to walk to and too expensive for me to take a cab.

Even though some changes have occurred in my life, I do my best not to let it get me down. Some people might start to think in terms of their ultimate demise, but I choose not to. I've come to despise the term "Bucket List." To me, it seems as though one is relatively near to their death. I'm not in denial, I know we will all die, but that seems morbid to me.

I instead have a never ending "to do" list. When I've completed a task, I just keep adding another to it. There's always something new that I can find to replace a completed task. This gives me a sense of living a long life.

Now, I'll move onto a very special point in my life. One friend who I did not mention in my prior chapter on friendships is my dear friend Allen O. Green. We met in January of 2010 through Facebook and although we had two gaps in our friendship; we've been great friends to this day. He has been the one person who I basically speak with every single day since we met. We even co-founded two Facebook groups. One is a Social issues group, and the other a Religious group.

While on the phone with him, he heard me have two seizures. And then while on Skype he witnessed me having another seizure. That must have been terrifying for him to not be able to do anything for me. However, the seizures did not last long before I was able to get back to speaking with him.

Allen has been there since 6 months after my initial brain surgery. He was the one who inspired me to continue with my writing after I wrote my first two articles. He was also the one who got me into blogging.

He is the reason that I completed this book. He kept encouraging me, giving me deadlines to complete certain chapters, and he helped me to get this book published.

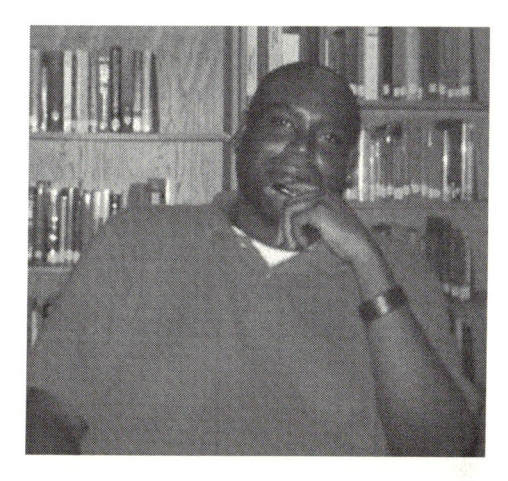

Allen

Also, one of my life time goals was to read the Bible from cover to cover. This I did in 2011. Whenever I was stuck on something that I did not understand, I turned to Allen for clarification. All in all, I consider him to be my very dearest friend.

So, what do I have in store for the future? I plan to devote time to my cancer page and my cancer group lending encouragement in any way I can. I hope to be able to write more articles for various magazines to get my message of hope and inspiration out to as many people as possible.

Speaking of hope, overall, the chance that a person will develop a malignant tumor of the brain or spinal cord in his or her lifetime is less than 1%. I would say that's a good thing in comparison to other types of cancers.

Now, onto what's new in adult brain tumor development. There is always research going on in that area. Scientists are looking for ways to prevent these types of tumors, and doctors are continuously working to improve the various methods of treatment.

One such development is in the area of imaging and techniques in surgery. One way is that patients drink a special dye a few hours before surgery. It glows when looking at it under the microscope with special lighting. This enables the surgeon to be able to better separate the tumor from the brain.

There are also tumor vaccines that are being tested to use against brain tumor cells. These vaccines are meant to treat the disease, not prevent it. The end goal is to stimulate the body's immune system to the tumors. In the end, I hope that they will find a cure not just for brain cancer, but for all cancers in general.

Now that I have mentioned what's new in brain cancer treatments, today if you were to pass me on the street, you would not think that I have a brain tumor, you would not think that I have seizures, and you would definitely not think that I have cancer. I would look like any other able bodied person. And I'm happy for this, because I want people to see me as Collette, since cancer does not define me, I define my cancer. I choose how significant a role it plays in my life. This reminds me of a book by Robert Buckman "Cancer is a word, not a sentence."

Ultimately, part of the cancerous tumor is still **in** my head, exploring around like a tourist in a foreign land.

Because of this, I likely won't ever be in remission - to which I say "so what!"

Regarding my cancer, I feel that the words of Ivan Noble, BBC Reporter fits best, "All the statistics in the world will not tell them what is going to happen to me, and I am grateful for the uncertainty and hope that provides."

Contact the Author

Email
collette@ettellocpublishing.com

Facebook Page
https://www.facebook.com/pages/Collette-Henry-Brain-Cancer-Awareness/138327939518298

Facebook Cancer Support Group
https://www.facebook.com/groups/304042236343729

Made in the USA
Charleston, SC
07 May 2013